Medi... Seniors Over 60

Step by Step Guide on How to Unlock the Full Power of Meditation to Deal with Everyday Life Challenges as A Senior Over 60

Introduction

Are you a senior over 60 who has decided to start taking proper care of your mind by meditating but now, well, now you have questions like:

- ***Where do I begin?***

- *How and where do I get started?*

- *Which basic meditation principles do I need to master to get gradually better at the practice?*

- ***How will meditation feel?***

- *What can I expect?*

- *Will it be harder to adopt now that I'm starting at an older age than most?*

All these are perfectly normal questions.

Fortunately for you, this book has the answers you need to start practicing meditation and make it a life-long habit. We'll cover pretty much everything about the subject:

- **What meditation is,**

- *What you need to know about the practice,*

- **Why you should meditate,**

- *How you should meditate, and a whole lot more.*

If you're still on the fence regarding meditation, this is the perfect resource to show you why meditation isn't a mere preference for seniors over 60; it is a necessity.

Read on to learn more.

PS: I'd like your feedback. If you are happy with this book, please leave a review on Amazon.

Please leave a review for this book on Amazon by visiting the page below:

https://amzn.to/2VMR5qr

Table of Content

Chapter 1: So, You Want to Start Meditating at 60+ Years Old?

Most people new to meditation find it weird to sit by themselves in silence, mulling over their inner-most thoughts, feelings, and sensations; to sit still and be content with doing nothing except soak in the tranquility around you — all of which, ironically, the mind resists. The older you start meditation, the more awkward the first days will likely be.

Meditation may seem strange at first, perhaps even intimidating to someone starting it a little later in life than most people, but that's alright. Humans have been practicing meditation for over 3,000 years, and most, if not all, have undoubtedly felt the same apprehension, dread, or awe you feel as you embark on your meditation journey.

Perhaps meditating is part of a larger personal development goal you would like to reach in a few years. Perhaps you want to start meditating because you want to be more focused, less reactive, or less anxious. Alternatively, perhaps you want to better your interpersonal ties, and you feel like meditation is just the thing that will ground you enough to make you a better, more relatable person.

Whatever your reason, training your mind via meditation is effectively awareness training. Awareness training can radically shift your outlook on life and improve it to extents hitherto unimagined. However, it calls on you to be consistent and make it as regular as brushing your teeth.

We experience our entire existence via our minds. Once you start meditating, your perspective on life will drastically change. You will start focusing more on the present and appreciate it for what it is, instead of burning a lot of mental energy each day fussing over things you'd like to do in the future or things you'd have liked to have done in the past.

However, getting motivated to begin meditating is not the same as really doing it. Too many people get hyped up to start meditation and do it for a week, only to let the motivational fire peter out and eventually drop the practice.

You will only reap the advantages of meditation if you begin and maintain a regular meditation practice. You must meditate regularly to start enjoying the benefits of meditation. As such, we might even say that you need less motivation to meditate and more discipline since the latter will allow you to do it regularly, whether you feel fired up for it or not.

Once you know what to do, you don't need to put in a lot of effort to learn to meditate and do it. Meditation is very easy to learn, and it only involves a few easy-to-do practices.

Let's get started by covering some practical matters and answering some of the most common questions regarding meditation, starting with what meditation is:

What Is Meditation?

Meditation is a series of techniques that promote heightened awareness and focused concentration. Meditation is a strategy for altering awareness by deliberately focusing your mind on the present instead of letting it wander, as is often the case. The deliberate focus provides various psychological advantages that we will cover deeply later.

At its most basic level:

Meditation is a mind-or-attention-training method, where you train your mind to stay focused on the present and what's happening at the moment, rather than letting it roam and latch onto the usual stream of steady, random thoughts.

Most of the time, our minds roam incessantly – we're worried, fantasizing, stressing, or mulling about the future or the past, etc. Meditation brings us back to the present moment and equips us with the tools we need to be less stressed, calmer, kinder, and more compassionate to ourselves and others.

Meditation is a form of attention/awareness training. It helps us take a step back from our distracted thoughts and return to the present in a clear and balanced manner.

Here are some important things that you need to know about meditation:

1. People have been meditating for thousands of years in numerous cultures worldwide.

2. Meditation has a long history in pretty much every religion, including Hinduism, Judaism, Buddhism, Christianity, and Islam.

3. Although meditation has a strong religious connotation, many people practice it regardless of their spiritual or religious views or practices.

4. Meditation is often utilized for psychotherapy, much more so today than in yesteryears.

5. There are numerous kinds of meditation.

Mindfulness

There are many different types of meditation. Every major religion has some form of contemplative meditation traditions embedded in them but this does not mean all meditation has religious connections – there also exists secular meditation techniques as well.

However, mindfulness meditation has grown in popularity in recent years more than any other kind of meditation, partly due to how simple, practical, and straightforward it is. Basic mindfulness meditation entails focusing on the present moment while remaining open-minded and nonjudgmental.

The goal of mindfulness meditation is not to cease your train of thought or empty your mind like some forms of meditation require you to do. Rather, the goal is to pay great attention to your thoughts, emotions and bodily sensations, so that you may see them more clearly without making assumptions or making up stories, as we're so often guilty of doing.

It is pretty simple and straightforward: All you need is to be present i.e. to be in the here and in the new where you allow your mind to get lost in the folds of fantasy —we've mentioned that the mind needs to stay open and that you should be nonjudgmental, but the problem with fantasy is that it plunges you into an unrealistic dream world and stops you from truly focusing on, and appreciating real, practical thoughts.

Simple as it is, mindfulness meditation can provide tremendous benefits with practice, including providing us better control over our behaviors and allowing us to be more kind and equanimous, even in stressful times. With enough practice, mindfulness meditation may even aid us to understand the causes of stress better give us insights on what to do to deal with it.

Though Buddhist practices are the primary origin of mindfulness meditation, today, you can find it offered as a completely secular practice that stresses factors like stress reduction, concentration cultivation, and the development of calmness and tranquility.

We need to clarify this because it's a common misperception that mindfulness is a religious practice. We also need to clarify that mindfulness meditation is a stress-reduction approach and a way to strengthen yourself mentally and give yourself greater control of your thoughts. It's also a form of self-care, as you will see in the next chapter.

Mindfulness is now gaining greater traction in professional settings, such as education, business, sports, and even the army/military, thanks to a growing body of studies demonstrating its demonstrable positive impacts on the human brain and body. This book will undoubtedly touch on a few of them as we learn more about the practice.

Mindfulness vs. Mindfulness Meditation

Though many often use the terms interchangeably, it's important to distinguish between mindfulness and meditation.

Mindfulness *is:*

The state/feeling of being fully lucid and switched on in the present moment without reflexive judgment, instinctive criticism, or mind-wandering/roaming.

On the other hand, mindfulness meditation **is *the practice of being fully present and aware in the present moment,*** which empowers us to be more aware throughout the day, especially in challenging situations where the mind is prone to roam and latch onto the past/future and unhelpful fantasies.

Mindfulness is the ability to be aware of what is happening presently without judgment. It is the practice of training one's attention to cultivate mindfulness.

Meditation is not limited to mindfulness meditation. For instance, transcendental meditation, which involves reciting a mantra to achieve a relaxed state of awareness, has become quite popular lately. It is a form of meditation that does not follow the tenets and ethos of mindfulness and mindfulness meditation.

However, in this book, we'll primarily concentrate on mindfulness and mindfulness meditation because it is the most popular and the easiest, most practical kind of meditation to master and practice, especially as an older adult new to meditation.

The Experience of Meditation (What It <u>MAY</u> feel Like)

When you close your eyes —if you choose to do so— and follow the meditation instructions in your first meditation session, you can expect your mind to wander, be easily distracted, and be quite restless.

Just because you have decided to sit and practice meditation does not mean you'll manage to sit and meditate smoothly right away, just as you wouldn't expect to tame a wild cat or horse overnight. And seeing as you're starting it in your older years, you may need a little more time to fully embrace it and warm your mind to take to it.

With this out of the way, meditation is a simple and uncomplicated process: all you need to do is sit and meditate. Just close your eyes (or not), concentrate on your breathing and allow your mind to work its magic.

You don't have to empty your mind to meditate or whatever else meditation 'gurus' insist you must do; just sit still and focus on the present stream of thought with an open-minded, nonjudgmental stance. However, do not fantasize. Meditation will be one of the few practices where you do not have/need to strive for anything – it's a state of tranquility that requires no effort.

There are no good or bad meditation techniques. Only awareness or non-consciousness exists, regardless of what all those experts try to tell you. Whenever you recognize you are lost in your thoughts and redirect your attention to the topic of emphasis (usually your breathing), that's meditation in practice. It isn't any deeper or more nuanced than this. All you have to do is constantly steer yourself back from distracting thinking to your breathing while maintaining your mindfulness. The time between lucidness/awareness and distracted thinking will get grow longer the more you practice.

Wrapping Up

The next chapter will focus on some truly impressive physical and mental benefits, most of which could be life-changing, especially at your advanced age. However, there is no guarantee that meditation will fix your issues or give you eternal happiness. Life, including all its difficulties and uncertainties, will continue happening as it has for millennia.

However, meditation can help you modify how you relate to, respond to, and assess events around you. It provides a haven of calm amid the mayhem outside. The transformation it brings about will be subtle, gradual, and ethereal yet ever so substantial with persistent practice. Meditation entails an increasingly heightened sense of knowledge and understanding that will completely revise how you feel about yourself, your environment, and those around you in the long run.

You now know what meditation is and what it entails. Let us now look at the benefits you'll get from the practice, benefits that could add a whole new dimension to your life as a senior.

Chapter 2: Top Physical & Mental Health Benefits of Meditation for Seniors

We all want to age gracefully —like fine wine, as people say, improving with each passing year. But we know – perhaps better than anybody else owing to our senior age – that this wish rarely ever comes true: aging brings its own set of losses and problems. Memory loss speeds up, digestion gets crankier and more difficult, aches and pains appear seemingly out of thin air, and our moods become less and less predictable.

The good news is that you have an array of things you can do right now that will help you get closer to that heralded objective of "aging gracefully, like fine wine."

One of these things is mindfulness meditation. As you will see from the content body below, regular meditation provides a wide array of mental and physical, not to mention emotional health advantages and benefits that should appeal to seniors.

Why Seniors (and All People) Should Meditate

Without further ado, let's look at the top benefits of meditation for seniors over 60 years of age:

Physical Health Benefits of Meditation for Seniors

The main physical health benefits related to meditation are:

#: Slowing down the progression of Alzheimer's & Dementia

Alzheimer's disease and common forms of dementia are chronic illnesses that commonly affect the elderly. Statisticians believe that up to half of all adults over age 85 in the US have dementia.

However, The National Institute on Aging (NIA) points out that "dementia is not a normal aspect of aging," contrary to what many people think.[1] More than enough people live well into their nineties and even the 100s without showing even the littlest signs and symptoms of dementia.

Dementia chips away at short and long-term memories, affects critical brain functioning, and can even lead to emotional devastation. However, combining breathing exercises and meditation can go a long way in helping reduce the progression of dementia-related disorders. Mindfulness meditation can help patients deal with the worry, stress, and sadness that

---

[1] https://www.nia.nih.gov/

frequently accompany the onset of memory loss.

#: Enhancing digestion

A range of factors, the most prevalent ones being nutrition and age, may alter our digestive functioning. Fortunately, it appears that meditation could be of significant help with digestion.

Meditation enhances circulation and boosts oxygen levels in your blood by encouraging deep breathing, which consequently helps improve digestion and make it smoother and more optimal.

Regular meditation can help if you're an older male or woman with digestive problems not brought about by other illnesses. However, meditation may not be enough if your digestion problems are because of some illness; you'll need to see a doctor about your issue.

#: Helping with the signs of menopause

Meditation can help with the symptoms of menopause, which is another later-life transition. Nina Bandoni, a blogger at "Sharing a Journey,"[2] a blog curation targeting older adults over age 50, began meditating well into her forties as she approached perimenopause. She says it has remained a constant in her life and helped with more than just menopausal symptoms.

"Meditation has helped me heal by connecting me a lot more profoundly to the deeper depths of my spirit and soul; it has helped guide my business practices and bolstered my intuition so that it's now sharper than it ever was," Bandoni says.

---

[2] https://sharingajourney.com/

"The majority of my yoga students have been ladies in their fifties and sixties. We all agree that it improves our lives as well as those of others around us," she continues.

Mental & Emotional Health Benefits of Meditation for Seniors

The starkest mental and emotional health benefits of meditation are:

#: Developing a lucid, sharp & focused mind

One of the many advantages of mindfulness meditation is its capacity to increase mental awareness and prevent cognitive decline —your physical brain structure changes because of regular meditation.

The amygdala, the brain part responsible for processing emotions like worry, stress, and anxiety, decreases, and parts tasked with personality development, self-awareness, and planning —like the prefrontal cortex— grow.

Because of this, meditators have better creativity, focus, and cognitive function, which can be especially beneficial to seniors facing the real prospect of cognitive ability and function deterioration.

#: **Managing moods and emotions**

Mood and emotion management is difficult for many of us, regardless of age. As we age, physiological changes tend to have an increasingly significant effect on mood stability and may make controlling our emotional reactions even more challenging.

It's no surprise that loneliness, melancholy, and even frustration and despair are common among us older folks, given the apparent difficulty that comes with adjusting and adapting to steadily losing our virility and independence and, often, the passing on of pets and people that are dear to us.

Meditation gives us the power to keep close tabs on our emotions and feelings without reacting or responding to them since it focuses on nonjudgmental presence.

Meditation also improves positive feelings and sentiments of wellness and empathy in young and older adults because the heightened awareness and nonjudgmental presence allow you to truly evaluate things and people and have an easier time viewing them from different perspectives.

#: Improving memory

Meditation stimulates the brain's memory centers. Improved cognitive function and memory are valuable allies, especially as we age because memory loss and deteriorating cognitive function are some of the more unwelcome "side effects" of advancing in age.

Mindfulness bolsters both long-and-short-term memory processes by improving awareness, lucidness, and blood circulation in the brain, thanks to mindfulness meditation's focus on deep breathing over a period regularly.

#: Promoting calmness and relaxation

We all need to take a break and simply breathe, especially as we get older and have already accomplished and done so much over the years. Everyone —regardless of age— benefits from taking time to chill out and smell some roses, go on a walk, or interact with loved ones.

Prescription medicines, despite their recommendation to older folks, cannot come close to matching the calming effect of mindfulness for elders. Meditation helps the elderly relax, better organize their thoughts, and maintain a crystal-clear perspective.

#: **Brings kindness and compassion**

Meditation makes you feel good about yourself. Meta, for instance, is a meditation type that focuses on and cultivates loving ideas and attitudes. You learn how to accept, forgive, and let go through such meditation practices.

To put it another way, the more work you put into meditation practices such as meta meditation, the more pleasant emotions you will have in life and the more pleasant you will be to those around you.

#: **Aids in the cessation of undesirable behaviors**

Meditation fosters the development of self-control and the cessation of addictions. Clinicians often use meditation to help with attention redirection, willpower, mood and impulse control, and understanding the roots of addiction, often with great success.

Patients can focus better on the present and away from their cravings. They can lift their mood and bolster their impulse control, which goes a long way in helping them combat intense cravings and stay away from relapses.

#: Sleep enhancement

Insomnia affects almost 50% of the entire US population. Meditation proficiency can aid in the control of unwanted thoughts that induce sleeplessness. Deliberately focusing your thoughts on the present or maintaining a nonjudgmental stance towards your stream of thought helps curb reactions to thoughts that may make it harder to sleep

Wrapping up

As your children start their own families, more friends, parents, relatives, and long-time friends pass away, or you struggle to transition from full-time employment to retirement, the weight of loss, sadness, and loneliness may become too much to bear.

Meditation provides room for peaceful thought and processing of these significant changes, allowing you to enter a new and inevitable life stage with grace and resiliency rather than stagnation and defeat.

You might find that as you gain more self-awareness through meditation, you become more capable of controlling your emotions and reactions. That is not to say that you will not feel the sting or pain of rejection, loss, or disappointment. You will feel them but also know exactly how to move forward and, more importantly, stay in motion once you have allowed yourself to experience the feelings surrounding them.

Practicing meditation and mindfulness leads to better decision-making. Better decision-making is important at this advanced life stage where decisions like caring for aging parents/allowing them to leave for advanced care in a nursing home, or moving locations to be closer to your grandchildren exert a heavy toll. Going about them properly, calculated, and groundedly is vital since they involve people you love very much.

Before we dive into how to practice meditation, let's discuss the basics and practicalities of meditation so that you know what is what before you start meditation. Chapter 3 examines these in considerable detail.

Chapter 3: The Basics & Practicalities of Meditation

Before you can learn how to drive, it is important that you first get acquainted with the steering wheel, gear shift, clutch, brake and acceleration pedals, windscreen wipers, side mirrors, etc. You also need to know what to do and the optimal driving position to be in so you can drive properly. Basically, you need to become familiar with the basics first.

The same applies to meditation: before you learn how to meditate, it is important to have the basics of the practice down pat so that once you begin to meditate, everything is much smoother, more coordinated, and hitch-free.

This chapter examines the most important basics and practicalities of the practice to make you more familiar with it and what you need to do.

1) Right time, right place

The first step is committing yourself to a steady, regular practice, preferably multiple times each week. Decide how much time you will set aside for meditation. For example, you can start with 15 or 20 minutes at first during which you will sit somewhere quiet (if at all there is noise, it should be very minimal).

Making a habit stick requires some discipline and persistence, so sticking to a schedule —the same time of the day, the same place — will greatly help you develop your meditation practice.

Many people stack meditation atop an already-established daily habit, such as daily morning/evening walks, teeth brushing, etc., to ensure they adhere to their meditation routine.

Morning meditation is the most common kind because most people find it easier to meditate early when their minds are at their clearest and distractions are at their fewest. However, you can meditate at any time you want, whether it's in the morning, afternoon, or evening.

2) What to wear

Put on whatever you want. The most vital thing here is that you're relaxed and comfortable. If you're wearing a belt, tie, or scarf, it's probably a good idea to loosen it first and remove any unpleasant, tight-fitting footwear or heels. You may also wear nothing if you like (though with this one, you need to be in a private place, preferably your own house).

3) How to sit

You can practice your meditation indoors or outdoors, on the floor, on a cushion, on a bench, on a chair, or anywhere else that suits you. You can safely ignore clichéd ideas of adopting a cross-legged position beside a tree or a slow-moving river —unless you want to do that.

As you get more and more comfortable with the practice, you may find it easier to meditate anywhere and with considerable distractions around you. However, at first, it is best to meditate indoors while sitting on a straight-backed chair. Sit upright, with your back pressed against the chair. This will help you maintain proper posture: neck relaxed, back straight, and chin ever-so-slightly slightly tucked in.

Place your hands gently on your knees or lap so that you're in a most comfortable position, which will make your meditation experience much more enjoyable.

4) Duration

The length of time you meditate will depend on your personal preferences, personal circumstances, and available time. The crucial thing to remember is that consistency takes precedence over the duration.

It's best to start with a brief 10-minute meditation session when you're initially starting, as it will be easier to follow. As you get more comfortable with meditation, you can increase the meditation period to 20 or 25 minutes.

If a 10-minute session seems a bit daunting when you first begin, try a 3-5-minute one instead. You will have an easier time of it the longer you practice mindfulness meditation.

5) Be clear on your motivation

People meditate for different reasons. As such, it is good to begin with an easily-discernible element of why you want to meditate before meditating.

If you merely have a vague idea of why you are doing it, you'll probably find it difficult to keep up with it. A clear idea of what you're looking to achieve out of meditation — whether it's to feel happier, calmer, more focused, or less stressed, for example — will go a long way toward establishing the correct mindset and staying committed to the practice.

6) Taking it day by day

Meditation is a lifelong journey, not a race to instant success. Take it one daily session at a time, remembering that this practice demands dedication, an endless pit of patience, and lots of practice, with the rewards only coming gradually.

There is no such thing as "good" or "poor" meditation, or "success" or "failure," only awareness or a lack of it — and distraction or a lack of it. That's all it boils down to, really. The more your mind learns to ignore distractions, and your awareness becomes bolstered, the easier meditation will become.

7) Staying mindful post-meditation

We meditate to improve our present-moment awareness. The goal of this practice is to help us be more aware of our surroundings and less likely to be distracted during the day. It's crucial to acknowledge the calm, undistracted state of your mind when you end your meditation session, and then make every effort to preserve this calm, lucid state of mind for the remainder of your day.

Make a clear plan for what you'll do after meditating, be it brushing your teeth, showering, or preparing breakfast. It's all too easy to complete a meditation session then laze around doing nothing, allowing the mind to wander again and, in so doing, losing the calm, quiet, expansive feeling achieved from meditating. Be careful, have a plan of activities to do after meditating, and make sure you carry this calmness and awareness into each subsequent activity.

With this covered, you are now ready to learn how to meditate and the various meditation techniques you can use to make the process much more flexible, adaptable, and enjoyable. Chapter 4 provides comprehensive coverage of this.

Chapter 4: How To Meditate Efficiently: A Step-by-Step Mindfulness Meditation Guide

When someone brings up meditation, it may conjure up thoughts of solitude and spirituality in your new-to-meditation mind – it may draw up images of peaceful, candlelight rooms in hallowed locations with soft background music.

However, meditation's greatest appeal is not that hallowed, tranquil allure associated with it. Rather, it's its simplicity, flexibility, and unparalleled accessibility. Its advantages are felt and enjoyed by folks of all ages, be they teenagers or 90-year-old ladies and gents, regardless of where they practice it, when they practice it and how they go about it.

The modern boomer's (yes, we make up the boomer generation) real-life stresses are certainly contributing to the sharp rise in popularity of this very ancient mind-body activity. Retirement, an empty nest, taking care of our old parents, chronic pain, and losing family and friends to disease or other causes are prime examples of tough life transitions we face as older folk.

Most, if not all, of these, are largely inevitable – they'll arrive eventually, and how well you're equipped to handle the stress and pressure determines how well you fare.

If you used to work full-time but are now retired —or if you used to keep yourself busy with your children's schedules but now have an empty nest and not a single kid in sight— the old techniques of distraction and engagement slowly get phased out until they are no longer practical.

Without the constant needs of kids or work to keep you engaged and focused, your thoughts may wander with increasing frequency to the past:

Was I a good, or perhaps parent? Did I put in enough hours? Why didn't I take more vacations and trips?

—or to future anxiety: What if I develop Alzheimer's disease? What happens if my money runs out? What if my grandchildren never come to see me? What if_

It is important to train yourself to focus on the NOW: focus on this new life chapter and be completely aware of —and very much conscious of— the present moment, instead of losing yourself to fruitless wanderings that will do little to nothing to improve your current situation. Meditation is perhaps the best strategy to achieve this level of lucidness, awareness, and acceptance.

The more you meditate, the more lucid and aware you will be. The more you will be able to acknowledge the present for what it is and enjoy it regardless of whatever life challenge or stressor comes your way.

Let's start with how to meditate.

How Do You Meditate?

Keeping the fundamentals covered in the previous chapter in mind, here is how to start a meditation practice.

NOTE: We need to emphasize that it is not necessary to make the process more complex than it needs to be. Unless you want these things, you don't need fancy mats, candles, robes, meditation stools, be outdoors, etc. All you need is yourself, a tranquil spot, and ten minutes of free time.

Here is how to perform a simple yet comprehensive mindfulness meditation routine focusing on your breathing. Fundamentally, this is the only kind of meditation you'll ever need. However, if you want to practice other kinds of meditation, you can also do it. But this one will be more than enough.

Without further ado:

1) Find a quiet, comfortable spot in your home, the backyard, or your favorite local park

Sit in a chair, put both feet up, or raise yourself up in bed with pillows—whatever position is most comfortable for you.

Because you'll be in this posture for a long time, experiment a little, at first, to see which positions lead to the least levels of discomfort. After a few minutes of experimenting, you'll settle on a position where you are most comfortable.

2) Establish a time limit

If you're just starting, a brief time limit, such as 5 or 10 minutes, may be beneficial for reasons we've already discussed. You can extend your meditation session the more familiar you become with the practice.

3) Pay attention to your body

You can be in a sitting position, with both feet on the ground, sit cross-legged, or kneel; any of these positions is okay. Simply ensure you are steady and comfortable and in an ideal position you can maintain for an extended time window.

4) Pay attention to your breathing

Follow the sensation of the breath as it gets into your lungs/body and leaves your body.

5) Recognize when your thoughts have wandered

Your attention will inevitably leave your breath and stray to other things. Simply pull your focus back to the breath when you notice you've wandered.

Please do not be too hard on yourself, even if your mind wanders for the entire 10 minutes session. Simply redirect your focus back to your breath and understand that the longer you meditate, the easier it will become to keep your mind from wandering.

6) Be gentle with your wandering thoughts

We must emphasize the point above – don't pass judgment on yourself, or obsess about the content of your wandering thoughts. Simply return to the point of focus —in this case, your breath.

7) End on a positive note

Don't just stop and stand up; begin by lifting your gaze gently when you are done (if you close your eyes when meditating, open them), and pause momentarily to listen to the sounds around you. Take note of how the body is currently feeling, and of your feelings and thoughts.

And that's it! That is all it involves. You don't need a hundred gimmicks and placebos to "meditate properly." Most of these are merely fancy additions added by 'gurus' so they can stand out in an increasingly competitive niche. All you need do to meditate is focus your attention on your breathing, pull back your attention when your mind wanders, and be kind to yourself when you slip up, as many times as is necessary.

Are you having trouble sitting still?

Walking meditation, often called "mindful walking," benefits the body and mind. *"Walking meditation links our body and mind,"* says Thich Nhat Hanh, a real Tibetan monk and a renowned Master of Zen and poet who founded the esteemed Engaged Buddhist movement.

"Breathing and walking are combined in walking meditation. You can take 2 or 3 steps as you breathe in, and then take 3, 4, or 5 steps when you exhale, and then you rinse and repeat."

While experts recommend 15 minutes of meditation for best results, starting small with 5- or 10-minute meditation sessions is fine and will give you all the benefits. Chapter 2 covered the benefits of meditation, and one of the benefits is that it staves dementia away.

Medical practitioners who use meditation on dementia patients usually do no more than 10-12-minute daily sessions with these patients, and the results are often very apparent in 12 weeks (12 minutes a day for 12 weeks.) As such, meditation does not have to be difficult or overly long to be beneficial.

Expanding Your Meditation Practices: A Few More Meditation Techniques for You

The purpose of meditating is to achieve a tranquil body and mind. Nevertheless, any difficulties you might have staying focused can have the opposite impact.

It could be that you do not fancy meditating while seated or that focusing on your breathing feels a tad monotonous or too bland for you, and you'd like to make it more interesting and engaging.

If this is your particular situation, here are a few more meditation techniques that will enhance your meditation process:

#1: *The Good Words Technique*

1. Think of a word or term that evokes a pleasant emotion in you, such as happiness, serenity, or any other pleasant emotion you would like to feel when meditating and after meditation.

2. Consider the meaning of that word. Use your fingertips to write it on your arm. Tap out the individual syllables on your palm or your forearm. Go with whatever you think will help keep this particular

word or term prominently in your thoughts.

3. Consider this emotive word or term as a color/hue, and visualize it in that particular color. It could be red, blue, purple, violet, etc. Then imagine a different color for that word's backdrop.

4. Continue to write the word on your palm or forearm, one syllable at a time, possibly even softly repeating the letters out loud.

5. Repeat for 10 minutes (set a timer so you can stay on track).

#2: The Body Scan Technique

The body scan entails progressively focusing on diverse feelings and body parts, from your head to your toes, rather than focusing your thoughts and attention on your breath, as in the basic mindfulness meditation routine outlined earlier.

1. Begin with the crown of your head. Bring your focus to the surface of the skin, inch by inch, slowly and thoughtfully. Check if you feel the scalp, the ears, the eyes, and the nose, and continue moving around your face, the ears, then down the neck and shoulders, then down to the toes, doing the same thing all through.

2. At first, it may feel like you are not feeling anything. However, as you keep at it, you may notice the onset of a whole new set of feelings. Some present sensations may be a mild warmth or feeling lightweight. You may also feel "neutral" sensations and feelings, such as itching or tingling. Some of them may even be unpleasant. For instance, you may have a sore spot on your feet.

3. Take note of any sensation you're having without judgment, and move whenever you need to relieve serious discomfort. Even if the experience is unpleasant, try not to respond by labeling it good or bad. Instead, simply acknowledge your emotions and then continue with your body scan.

4. And of course, just like before, if you realize that your mind has strayed, simply ease your attention back to your body and continue with the body scan.

#3: The Mindful Eating Technique

Mindful eating is another useful technique to attempt.

Make the necessary time, not to mention space, so you can give this experience your complete attention, rather than just chowing down on whatever meal is on your menu.

You can practice this one whenever you're alone and eating a meal. Alternatively, you can set aside some time to practice mindful eating with a basic item like an apple or a raisin.

Mindful eating is often a beneficial (and fun) exercise that may open up a new universe of exciting sensory experiences; it has shown the capacity to improve weight loss. Have you noticed that you tend to eat less when you pay close attention to how hungry you are, what you eat, and how you're eating? Practicing this technique will inevitably lead you to eat less, making it easier to watch your calorie intake and lose weight more easily.

1. Take note of every detail of your eating experience and your particular reactions. As you take your seat and prepare to eat, pay attention to how you feel at that moment, just before you eat. Are you starving? Is your stomach grumbling?

2. Examine the food carefully. How does it look? Now examine it thoroughly: Is it hot or chilly outside? What is its aroma? When you hold it, does it —say— make a mushy sound?

3. Focus on your reactions as you prepare to put the first spoonful in your mind. More drooling? Are you thinking of your next bite already?

4. What happens when food reaches your tongue? Take note of the mounting desire to chew on it. Are you ready to swallow and go on to the next bite?

5. What happens to the texture of the meal as you chew? What does the food feel like as it passes from your mouth and down your throat? Do you have any sensations in your stomach?

6. Please do not rush the process. Take your time. Move on to your next

mouthful after finishing the previous one, taking note of everything about this experience, from the aromas, tastes, and physical sensations to your inner desires, feelings, and impulses.

Meditating the Right Way

Setting aside some time for meditation is crucial for developing a pattern and being comfortable with it. Even a few minutes per day can have a significant impact.

Some people resent having to take time out of their busy days; it could be that you have other things to do or other things you could enjoy more doing. However, consistent meditation is essential. It's a valuable practice for returning to the present moment, and it will especially go a long in stressful or high-pressure situations.

You must also understand that when you stop meditating, you should not cease being mindful. Carrying this mindfulness into every activity following your meditation session will greatly benefit you. The goal of mindfulness meditation is for us to become more conscious in all aspects of our lives, not simply while sitting on a chair or our specially designated meditation cushion. The goal is to make mindfulness, awareness, and calm a practical, oft-used element in our day-to-day lives.

While mindfulness meditation is certainly not about letting your mind wander, it is also not about attempting to clear your mind, as it is with some forms of meditation.

The tricky issue with meditation practices that involve trying to empty your mind is that this is often really difficult to achieve, let alone sustain for 10 minutes or more, as it is second nature for your brain to latch onto thoughts and wander. Instead, this practice entails paying attention to whatever is going on, in and around you, in the present moment, particularly our inner thoughts, feelings, and sensations.

Though self-meditation is an important aspect of a comprehensive practice, you may find that a meditation tutor will help make the process a lot more streamlined and easier to do. The steady supervision of a seasoned tutor can be quite beneficial, especially to beginners, because a beginner's mind tends to wander easily, and a teacher's prompt, straightforward directions can help us return quicker to the present moment.

When the Mind Wanders...

We cannot emphasize this point enough:

We've brought it up several times and provided brief one-liners on what to do when your mind wanders. Here, we examine the issue a little more comprehensively:

Mind-wandering is unavoidable: let that sink in, then accept it for what it is: a meditation fact.

The mind is a natural wanderlust. Thus:

Your thoughts will inevitably wander during meditation. Other feelings in your body, events occurring around you, simply being lost in your own thoughts, fantasizing about the present, past, or future, possibly criticizing yourself or other people around you, etc., are all mind-wandering possibilities. And this is perfectly normal; thinking is just as natural as breathing.

Simply observe what you are/were thinking about or what is/was distracting you when this happens, then pause for a bit.

You don't have to take immediate action to return your focus to your breath. Instead, let go of whatever you are/were thinking about, re-open your focus, and slowly bring your awareness back to your breath, making sure to be present for every inhalation and expiration.

Don't merely bring your attention back to your breathing. Reset by taking a moment to pause, re-open your focus, then gently return and focus on your breath.

The mind will invariably stray again after a few breaths. When it does, please don't be too hard on yourself. Instead, remind yourself that all this, the **mind wandering** <then> **noticing it when it happens** <then> **refocusing** <then> **noticing when the mind wanders again and refocusing** is natural, and how you meditate and practice mindfulness as a daily habit. What matters is how we react when it occurs.

Simply acknowledge the particular thoughts distracting you — without passing judgment on them or allowing them to drag your focus and attention away completely — and take a minute to return to the present moment and resume meditation.

The practice of "coming back" is where we develop our meditation skills and habituate mindfulness. **Coming back, time after time**. Notice it — think about it— then pause before returning to the present. By and by, meditation will become easier, and distractions will be fewer and farther between.

You now know how to meditate and what to do to make the process smooth. You understand how to transition back to awareness and meditation when your mind inevitably wanders.

Next up, we shall look at something that afflicts the elderly at such a high rate, owing to their numerous experiences and inevitable traumas and losses – PTSD–. We shall especially focus on how meditation is a godsend that fosters healing from this stress disorder and helps us work towards being happier, more peaceful versions of ourselves.

Chapter 5: Meditation–A Phenomenal Way to Heal from Post-Traumatic Stress Disorder

While the past decade has seen numerous programs, rehab ventures, and structures put in place to curb Post-Traumatic Stress Disorder over the years, it's unfortunate that not enough of these have been specific to seniors and older folks.

It is applaudable that so much effort has gone into setting up solid PTSD structures and programs for war vets and other PTSD-afflicted persons that other areas have born the brunt of it all. All too often, seniors are on the receiving end of the short end of the stick in the effort against PTSD, which has left far too many of us grappling with the issue on our own and suffering the mental and emotional issues that stem from it.

As seniors, we have the blessing of having lived more years and having seen more than most people around us. However, we also have the curse of having experienced more bad things and occurrences than most people around us. We've undoubtedly lost more friends and loved ones, endured more trauma, had more unpleasant experiences, etc., than most of our younger counterparts. We also grew up in an era that didn't emphasize mental and emotional health – at least compared to today – and thus, any trauma that we may have suffered in years gone may not have been sufficiently taken care of.

Meditation can help seniors suffering from post-traumatic stress disorder. If you have taken an extra step and started to get therapy, you should know that while meditation will substitute their medications, it can help you recoup mental health stability faster and help with keeping calm. There is also no need to attend a formal meditation class; you can do it from the comfort of your home.

What Qualifies as Trauma, and How Does It Affect our Brain Structure?

Before we get into what trauma is, it is necessary to point out that meditation can aid in the recovery from PTSD and trauma. However, it isn't necessarily the silver bullet/panacea we may hope for it to be.

Meditating will not instantly make past trauma vanish. Meditation could exacerbate trauma, owing to the nonjudgmental examination of thoughts going through your mind, some of which may be rooted in traumatic events in your past.

Meditation makes the activity in the brain more conscious and deliberate. Still, we are not always ready to be present with what we perceive and examine in our minds, especially when it relates to traumatic thoughts and happenings from our past. As such, trauma-informed meditation considers the possibility of re-traumatization via mindfulness and takes precautions to guarantee that meditation gets to heal and build your mind without adding to the damage.

What is trauma? Trauma is only definable by the person who has gone through it. That's it. There is no single event or a specific set of circumstances that constitutes trauma.

The American Psychological Association defines trauma as *"an emotional reaction/response to any/every incident that the experiencer considers to be deeply disturbing or significant."* What may be deeply traumatic to someone else may be little more than a source of endless jokes and hilarity for you, and vice versa.

Trauma causes psychological harm and completely transforms the physiological brain structure. Neuroplasticity —the changing/transformation of the brain structure— often praised as a favorable trait in humans, could have negative and positive effects. For example, the plasticity/malleability that causes our brains to change in reaction to trauma also allows us to heal.

Meditation aids trauma recovery by providing a fresh perspective on past and present events, altering our brain structure, and effectively setting the gears of neuroplasticity in motion, thus helping reverse the damage and heal your mind.

Let us get into how meditation helps heal trauma some more:

How Meditation Heals Trauma

Meditation aids in the separation of our emotions, thoughts, and sense of self. Via meditation, we learn that we're not our feelings/emotions and thoughts and that not all of our thoughts are valid or worthy of a response.

We may apply these similar concepts to our particular manifestations of trauma with constant practice. We can break free from compulsive reactions and trauma-related anguish by approaching traumatic expressions in the mind and body with an attitude of curiosity and compassion instead of fear, anxiety, and revulsion.

Traumatic stress causes damage to your hippocampus and prefrontal cortex and increases activity in your amygdala, which controls our automated freeze-fight-flight response. Meditation has the opposite effect on these very same brain regions. It increases activity in our hippocampus and prefrontal cortex while decreasing amygdala hyperactivity, thereby helping greatly with healing from trauma and PTSD.

However, we need to reemphasize that while meditation certainly can help us recover from trauma, total recovery is not always straightforward. Trauma survivors may have ignored thoughts, body sensations, or emotions associated with prior trauma for a long time. Closing your eyes to tune inward might trigger flashbacks and extreme re-traumatization or hyperarousal when trauma is present. Meditation may, in such cases, appear to exacerbate your trauma.

Traumatic energy tends to remain in your body and mind until it's recognized and promptly released with love and compassion. This is a technique that almost all psychotherapists use to help with trauma and PTSD. Meditation can also help with this, albeit it is not a one-size-fits-all approach.

If meditation agitates rather than calms you, it is not a personal failure on your part, and neither is it because you're doing it wrong. In such an instance, it will do you a lot of good to seek professional therapy that can help you untangle the traumatic events that keep bogging you down so that meditation can start calming you instead of making your trauma flare-up.

5 Tips and Strategies for Meditation as a Trauma/PTSD-Healing Tool

Here are a few more invaluable tips on how to make meditation work effectively as a PTSD-healing tool below:

1) Consult a licensed trauma-informed expert in meditation

Some meditation tutors may neglect the trauma experience of pupils, and not nearly every trauma therapist knows how to teach meditation for effective trauma healing. Finding a guide who comprehends both is essential for incorporating meditation into the trauma recovery approach.

When meditation gets overwhelming, a trauma-informed meditation expert may suggest tools, tips, and strategies you can lean on so that your meditation practice feels and IS actually safe and successful.

2) Stay within your particular tolerance window

Each of us has a particular tolerance window, a range of arousal within which we can perform efficiently.

Trauma survivors may have limited introspection and/or body awareness capacity before uncontrollable mental anguish kicks in compared to other people who haven't dealt with trauma. Recognizing when you are stretching the limits of your particular tolerance window and knowing how to get grounded again safely are all part of trauma-informed mindfulness.

3) Meditate in a secure environment

A simple directive, such as "close your eyes," can sometimes drive you out of your comfort zone if you're a trauma survivor.

Meditation provides a secure mental environment in which to engage with powerful or challenging emotions and thoughts, but practicing your meditation in an insecure, uncomfortable physical location can quickly negate that value. You need to match the secure mental environment that meditation provides you with a secure physical environment.

Large groups of people, the outdoors, schools, hospitals, or any environment associated with the root of our trauma can all make us feel uncomfortable and thus negate any benefits that meditation could bring us.

4) Practice love, compassion, and tolerance with yourself

Meditation is not a linear process that becomes easier with each session, nor does it cure trauma overnight.

Trauma profoundly impacts our minds and bodies, and while we can recover, recovery takes time. Self-compassion and patience are virtues we can develop in certain meditation routines. However, they are qualities we must apply to all meditations and the general healing process. Remember that the kinder you are to yourself, the more your self-esteem grows, and the easier healing will become.

5) Meditation is only but one cog in a comprehensive set of recovery tools

Meditation is an excellent tool for linking us to that calm, stable mental state that we all know exists, regardless of our history or present circumstances. However, if you've experienced trauma in the past, meditation may be most effective when combined with a holistic, professionally-guided, integrative healing approach overseen by a trauma expert. If you have had traumatic experiences in your past and are perhaps struggling with PTSD, reach out to a licensed therapist. The combination of professional help and regular, steady meditation will do wonders for your mental health.

Next up, we look at apps, podcasts, websites, and other digital resources that will help you get started faster and make your meditation practice streamlined, smoother, and more enjoyable long-term.

Chapter 6: Top Meditation Apps, Podcasts, and Websites to Get Your Started

Apps, podcasts, and websites are excellent resources for meditation —if we're being honest, they are also excellent resources for most other things.

As a senior gentleman or lady, you are probably overly enthusiastic about computers, software, podcasts, and apps. But in truth, the digital world is so easy to get into and navigate these days that just about anyone can delve into and gain from it with little to no problems, even without prior computer education and savviness.

This chapter looks at several digital resources – with apps being the most prominent – that will help improve and streamline your meditation practice. The more you use these apps and digital resources, the easier and more fun your experience with meditation will become.

Without further ado, here are the top apps, websites, and podcasts for meditation:

1: Headspace

The Headspace app is accessible on both Android and iPhone. The first ten sessions are free when you join up. After that, you can have limitless meditation sessions for a monthly charge. You may also use the app to track your meditation progress and assess your achievements as you get on with your meditation journey.

2: Soundrown

The free songs and tracks for instant listening available through this website —most of which are also available on SoundCloud— offer focus-friendly sounds on demand, helping weed out the aural distractions that often contribute to mind wandering (or negative, spiraling) thoughts.

3) Calm

The immensely popular Calm app, which focuses on obtaining better sleep and reducing stress, provides a great foundation for mindfulness newbies.

Over a hundred guided meditations are available, as well as a unique "sleep stories" feature in which soothing tales [are] recounted by well-known voice actors to help you relax and fall asleep.

4: Tara Brach's Guided Meditations

We'll name-drop Tara Brach a few times in the chapters below because of her extensive meditation research work. Tara Brach's website and the accompanying podcast may pique your curiosity if you feel interested in ancient spiritual meditation influences.

Brach is the creator of a meditation center in Washington, DC, one of the country's largest, and she wisely mixes her psychotherapy background with apt Buddhist teachings.

5: The Meditation Podcast

The Meditation Podcast, hosted by Jeane and Jesse Stern, provides "easy, basic meditations" for anyone "living with an emotional or health difficulty."

Many listeners have provided deep testimony about how the podcast has helped them deal with physical and mental health issues such as anxiety, strokes, and emotional loss. The podcast utilizes tranquil audio tones that regulate brain waves and bring forth a state of peace and calmness, aiding relaxation.

6: Guided Meditation for Beginners on YouTube

After typing the exact-match keywords "Guided Meditation for Beginners" on the YouTube search tab, you'll get hundreds of results. Choose one that appeals to you visually, in terms of approach, tracks, and music, and, certainly, the meditation instructor/guide in the video: The more committed and invested you are, the more successful you will be.

7: The Muse Headband

For real-time neurofeedback, Mark Levine, the app's proprietor, proposes utilizing the Muse headband in tandem with the "Ten Percent Happier" app. Dan Harris, the co-founder of this latter app, also wrote the book "Meditation for Fidgety Skeptics."

Levine recommends this book to all his meditation coaching clients and customers who're just starting meditation and would like to fast-track their adoption process so that it becomes a regular habit in the shortest time possible.

Speaking of turning meditation into a regular habit that you get to practice over a long time without forgetting or constantly putting it off, the next chapter comprehensively examines how you can make the habit stick to ensure you can enjoy its benefits for many years to follow.

Chapter 7: Making Meditation A Life-Long Habit–10 Tips to Make Meditation a Daily Habit

It's usually relatively easy to begin something new - an exercise routine, a new diet, a new hobby interest. However, keeping at it and making sure you keep doing it past the first two weeks can be difficult. The initial excitement inevitably fades. The novelty eventually wears off.

This problem is atypical to meditation, especially when the activities become monotonous (and they will become monotonous since you'll repeat most of the things you'll be doing each session.) It's important to remember that we're teaching the mind to change how we perceive and relate to our feelings and thoughts, which requires time, persistence, and discipline.

Frustration with the mind's refusal to "empty" or "clear" is a primary reason so many people give up on meditation. Going in, it is crucial to understand that your mind will always latch onto thoughts since this is what it's trained to do. Meditation will not miraculously stop thoughts flowing in. all it'll teach you is how to take a step back and watch thought objectively, without judgment.

Allowing thoughts to arrive and go with an objective, accepting state of mind is the primary goal here. It's a skill that requires studying, honing, and perfection. And the only way to master this ability is to make meditation a habit.

The more you practice meditation, the more benefits you'll experience. The more benefits you experience, the more you'll understand how the mind feels and thinks. The more this happens, the more you'll feel driven to take active steps toward a happier, healthier life –

one filled with more clarity, serenity, satisfaction, and compassion.

Chris Penhall, an author, producer for the BBC, and a staunch advocate for meditation, says this:

"I first learned about Headspace —↕an app we covered in the previous chapter— about a year ago, at the start of 2021. I was doubtful at first, but I believed anything that had the potential to help me deal with my continual fear and stress was worth a shot.

"One year later, I've completed 365 consecutive days of meditation with Headspace. I've reduced my therapy sessions as my therapist, and I have concluded that my recovery has progressed to the point where fewer sessions will do. At the very least, I'm a little better at extracting myself from self-destructive spirals since tapering off the meds.

I'm not free of anxiety, but I'm more prepared to handle it now. The difficult thing, like any other habit, is staying with it."

Chris Penhall is 66 years old.

Here are some pointers to consider if you want to make this practice a daily one:

1) Choose a realistic amount of time

Chris Penhall says,

"I used to believe that meditation entailed sitting in silence for hours. But I found that setting a brief, attainable objective made me likelier to stick with it. I settled on 20 minutes. I barely did 10 minutes some days, but I never pushed myself to meditate beyond 20."

2) Do it first thing in the morning

Mark Levine, whom we mentioned and linked to in the previous chapter, says:

"While this may not necessarily be the case for everyone, we have the most control over our time in the morning. It also puts you in a good mood for the rest of the day.

If the mornings aren't convenient for you, I'd suggest setting up a definite period each day—perhaps your lunch break. You can change it up now and again, but meditating as part of your everyday routine is quite beneficial."

3) Do it anywhere and everywhere

You don't get sweaty exercising the mind as you do your body. So, you can comfortably meditate in your regular clothing, wherever you are, and go on with your day without a hitch.

Here are some locations you can meditate in whenever you find yourself in them:

- Aboard a city bus

- In a chair in your apartment

- On a subway train, while standing

- In the park

- On flights

- In hotel rooms, while traveling

- In your car, while in traffic

- At work, in a quiet spot.

- IAtn a party, perhaps in the restroom

- Waiting in line at the DMV

Mark Levine is a huge proponent of meditating "anywhere and everywhere:"

"I used to believe that I needed a peaceful area to meditate. But I discovered that it was possible to practice in any place if the noise was steady—that is, noise that didn't change and that I could shut out.

I once meditated across the street from a Baptist preacher preaching through a megaphone on a Sunday morning. My first reaction was to recoil and think to myself, "This is ruining my meditation!" But then, I noticed that his speech was muffled by the megaphone, much like the voices in those old-school Charlie Brown cartoons.

I was able to shut out the voice and continue meditating after I realized that it was another extension of my immediate environment. However, if you are surrounded by people having random exchanges, you should consider going somewhere else."

4) Bring a Positive Attitude

Approach meditation with a positive mindset. Relax, be curious, and be friendly. Maintaining awareness of these attributes will benefit you as you navigate the ups and inevitable downs of meditation —and they're many.

Take some deep breaths, and let yourself relax and be at peace with yourself and your environment if you feel yourself straining too hard or criticizing yourself. Remember that the goal of meditation is not to gain full mental control or completely stop thinking. The goal is to approach whatever happens with more compassion, serenity, and acceptance.

Tara Brach, whom we covered and linked in the previous chapter, says:

"There needs to be nonjudgmental, open, and allowing calmness and presence in order to observe clearly what is in that present moment. Do not criticize or praise – merely observe and assess."

5) Manage Your Expectations

"Even if it is not always easy to do, mindfulness meditation is really simple and straightforward. It necessitates a dedication beyond everything else. "Admiring the "idea"

of meditation doesn't really achieve anything," Sharon Salzberg, a mindfulness meditation teacher for over 40 years, states.

"You need to actively meditate, no matter how much you stumble in the beginning. It's very important that you make it a regular habit that you're accustomed to as quickly as possible."

Remember that meditation and mindfulness aren't cure-alls. Mind-wandering will not just go away. Difficult thoughts and emotions related to past traumatic events may surface. It may seem a little too challenging to keep your focus present on your breath when you first begin meditating, especially early on. But it'll get easier with time; this is for sure.

First, assess how it feels to be in the present moment before attempting to push the envelope and perhaps arrive at an out-of-body experience, which some veteran meditators can do. Observe your thoughts, emotions, and physical sensations.

Ms. Tara Brach says: *"The ideal thing with this is to be present and aware of what is going on. Just that. The rest is secondary. Set all expectations and judgments about what will happen aside."*

6) Maintain your streak

Chris Penhall says that staying consistent and keeping her streak alive (yes, this Chris is a she) was integral in making meditation a habit in her life:

"This was the most important component in keeping my daily habit going. I didn't want to disrupt my daily meditation streak after I committed.

The Headspace app includes small badges that show how far you've come: One day, three days, ten days, fifteen days, thirty days, and ninety days. 180 days. 365 days. This was a tremendous incentive for me. I'd take note of my streak number after every session. This created a beneficial feedback loop. I would meditate, check my streak count, and be pleased with myself for making progress."

Your streak is your ally in making meditation a true habit. Keep it alive at all costs.

7) Scale back when necessary

Chris Penhall says:

"I couldn't always complete my 20-minute session. Sometimes, I was unwell, traveling, or lacked sufficient energy to meditate. I'd perform a briefer-than-usual session on such days. I'd practice meditation for, say, half the usual duration, simply doing the basics: taking deep breaths, tuning in to my senses and body, and tacking the in-out rhythm of my breathing."

Being nice to yourself is an important aspect of overcoming anxiety, so don't be too hard on yourself if you fail to stick to your meditation plan. Just do the bare minimum to keep the streak active, then pick it up again tomorrow.

8) Accept that you won't be perfect

"I'm bad at this," "My mind isn't wired for meditation," etc., are all things you're bound to think, especially in the first few days when you're only getting familiar with meditation, and your mind keeps wondering. However, motivate and discipline yourself to keep at it. Meditation requires repetition. It's an exercise. It's also acceptable to make mistakes during training.

If the mind keeps wandering, you should halt, take note of your source of distraction, and then let it go. Mark Levine says:

"When I originally attempted to meditate, I became enraged every time I noticed myself

wandering and latching on to random trains of thought. I would think, "Damn!"My mind is wandering uncontrollably. I'm awful at meditation."

The thing to do is to realize you're distracted, take note of your source of distraction, and then reset and get back to it. This way, each time you make a mistake, you give yourself a chance to progress and improve by evaluating distractions and noting which ones recur most often. It's like learning to ride a bicycle – If you are not hitting the ground and having to pick yourself off the floor, you are not learning.

9) Make your meditation about those around you

Mark Levine says:

"Meditation is often thought to be very self-centered. However, by looking after my own mental health, I've been more willing to treat

others properly. Acceptance, empathy, and patience are traits that will greatly aid those whom you love and care about. If you're not necessarily inspired to practice meditation for yourself, keep in mind that it may benefit those around you and make their lives better."

10) Remember, meditation is not magic

Meditation is an awesome mind training tool, but it isn't a panacea or some sort of silver bullet. Tara Brach says,

"I still had anxiety, stress, and melancholy on occasion. I'd get caught up in a negative cycle and say to myself, "This is not fair" Every day, I meditate" (As is all too apparent, there's always an opportunity for improvement, both in meditating and living in general.)

"The argument is that anxiety and stress are natural parts of life. Meditation will not make

them go away. But it offers me the requisite tools to instantly recognize and deal with those feelings and sentiments when they emerge in a constructive, healthy manner."

Bonus Tip: Enjoy the journey

Meditation isn't something you practice for a year, two years, or five years and then consider yourself "cured" It's something you practice continuously and improve on for the rest of your life. So, rather than anticipating how you'll feel later, try to appreciate your sessions for what they are now: brief periods of calm and stillness where you get to disconnect from the chaos of your daily life.

Mark Levine says:

"I began meditating, believing myself to be an anxious individual. But I've since discovered that identity isn't that fixed. I'm but a mere man that has anxiety from time to time. It doesn't make me an anxious man.

And, owing to meditation, I am far more capable of dealing with those emotions than I ever was previously. I'm only at the start of my adventure, and there's a lot more intensive learning (and going off the rails, from time to time) ahead of me."

Coax yourself back to mindfulness a thousand times as if you were training your puppy. You will progressively learn to relax and get centered with the breath over weeks (even months) of practice. This process will go through several cycles, with stormy days that alternate with clear, hitch-free days. Just keep going. As you practice mindfulness on your breath, you'll notice that it helps you connect with and calm your entire mind and body.

With all this in mind, the next chapter examines the challenges of taking up meditation as a senior and how you can overcome them to meditate with minimal problems.

Chapter 8: The Challenges of Taking Up Meditation as a Senior & How to Overcome Them

Meditation appears straightforward, but it can be incredibly challenging. Running into numerous challenges and stumbling incessantly, especially in the first two weeks of meditation, does not mean you are failing at it, are awful at meditation, or that meditation perhaps "isn't meant for you."

It's natural to experience setbacks whenever you start meditating. These setbacks could be in the form of general resistance, overload, anxiety, fear, boredom or restlessness. These should not stop you though, as these hurdles will pass with time and consistent practice. In the end, you will find it easier to meditate.

It's important to understand that everyone approaches meditation with a 60+-year-old lifetime of training. Your mind has grown occupied to being occupied. It hasn't grown used to being still. So, it will buck and kick until it becomes used to the strange concept of letting go, staying calm, and not doing anything for 10-20 minutes.

Here are the most prevalent obstacles and hurdles of meditating and how you can navigate them, so your meditation process is smoother:

Obstacle 1: Finding Time to Meditate

Finding time to be by yourself and meditate daily is the most common challenge, but it shouldn't truly matter if you go a day or three without meditating.

The most beneficial practice is certainly one that's repeated regularly, but what matters most is that you pick up where you left off and devote ten or fifteen minutes — or whatever time you choose — to mind training.

If it has been a while since you've meditated, say, a month, it would be best to start with the basics of meditation afresh. This will ensure you don't experience 'teething' difficulties when you resume.

Obstacle 2: Feeling Sleepy

It's common to feel drowsy — and perhaps nod off — when you first start practicing meditation, especially at this age. This is due to the mind's conflation of "doing nothing" with rest. It will eventually recognize the difference, subtle as it may be at first, between the relaxed focus (what you are aiming for) and complete relaxation (which is the kind you have when sleeping).

Here are three suggestions that may help you stay attentive and awake:

1. Do your meditation sitting up, not lying on your back/side.

2. Try meditation early, preferably first thing in the morning, while your mind is fresh.

3. Allow some fresh air in by opening a window.

Obstacle 3: Too Many External Distractions

Many beginners feel that every session should begin with dead silence, something that makes them too sensitive to distracting sounds and other distractions. Understand that meditation does not necessarily ask you to sit in complete silence. Rather, the purpose is to "settle into being" one with your surroundings. Be one with all of the sounds, chirps, and little elements of turbulence that come with them, whether it's a noisy neighbor who likes to raise their voice from time to time, screaming kids playing outside your home, or a truck reversing.

Let those sounds come and go without resistance or judgment, rather than fixating on them or actively trying to ignore or tune them out, then becoming frustrated when your efforts are futile. If you're having trouble with this at first, you can always use earplugs at first, or noise-canceling earbuds.

Obstacle 4: Restlessness

Meditation can initially feel tedious since we are so used to being active. If this is the case, focus on extremely particular sensations, such as the out-breath. You could also try to manage your breathing by inhaling deeply and then exhaling slowly; this has the automatic effect of calming you down and diminishing your restlessness.

Above all, try not to be too harsh on yourself when you stumble or are too restless to meditate for more than a couple of minutes without going off the rails. Simply use the advice this book has already given you and reset as many times as possible, without resistance, making sure to keep a nonjudgmental stance.

Obstacle 5: Self-Criticism

It's all too easy to criticize ourselves when we first start meditating:

"I'm making too many mistakes! I'm really awful at this! I will never really be able to properly focus on and keep track of my breath! I can't keep my mind clear!"

Almost everyone who's tried to meditate has had some level of self-criticism and self-doubt, especially in the beginning. Although this inborn instinct is partially responsible for the evolution of man (self-criticism/self-doubt led to fewer unnecessary risks, which helped humans live longer and pass their genes to future generations), it is not beneficial in this case.

Remember that the goal of meditation is not to achieve bliss, halt your train of thought, or have the perfect, tranquil meditation experience; it's simply being present and okay with whatever is going on at the time. Try to discard any/all preconceived notions about what constitutes good, terrible meditation, or whether —or not— you've accomplished something/anything: just meditate.

We all possess the capacity to be clear, calm, and mindful, regardless of external distractions, the popping up of random thoughts, the environment not being ideal, etc.

Obstacle 6: Pain

When you start meditating for longer sessions as a senior, you may experience aches resulting from sitting/holding your meditation position for an extended time. It might be a dull cramp or ache in your back or a sudden, transient pang in the legs.

At first, when the aches are mild, try just to take note of them and accept whatever it is. Recognize that it is a sensation, just like every other one you experience, and that it will pass. If the ache persists or worsens, try focusing on a different portion of your body to take your mind off the pain. You can as well adjust and tweak your meditation position as necessary, especially if the discomfort/pain becomes unbearable.

Obstacle 7: Fear

Fear or panic may set in on uncommon occasions when meditating. For instance, your train of thought may roll on to past trauma experiences, which may lead to anxiety or fear (we've already covered this.) If this happens, attempt to focus on something other than your body. You could focus on the air you're inhaling and exhaling or on external sounds around you.

Try not to get too fixated on whatever thing is causing emotional distress, be it your thoughts/memories or something in your immediate environment. If it becomes too intense, do not be afraid to open your eyes (if you meditate with your eyes closed) or take a three-minute break from meditation before resuming.

Conclusion

By now, you've learned a lot about meditation for seniors:

- *The importance of meditating*

- *How to meditate properly*

- *How to navigate the inevitable obstacles when you start meditating —not to mention tons of other interesting things about meditation.*

If you implement what you've learned and use the tips and strategies provided, you'll be able to meditate better and enjoy the process more and more, making it easier to make meditation a life-long habit.

Once you make meditation habitual, you'll enjoy the full benefits of meditation. For example, you'll find it easier to be calmer, more composed, and more objective. You'll cope with hardship and tough times better, owing to your consistent mind training, among many other things. You'll find that your life will improve in ways you couldn't have fathomed.

PS: I'd like your feedback. If you are happy with this book, please leave a review on Amazon.

Please leave a review for this book on Amazon by visiting the page below:

https://amzn.to/2VMR5qr

Made in the USA
Las Vegas, NV
14 February 2025